THIS PRACTICE JOURNAL BELONGS TO:

Name: _____

Address: _____
_____
_____
_____

Phone #: _____

Email: _____

If found, please return. As a reward? Good Karma :)

YOGA PRACTICE

Journal

This journal is a simple way for you to log your learning, track your progress, and document your journey as a yoga teacher. The best teachers are always the best students, and at YOGABODY, we believe practice is everything.

WELCOME TO YOGABODY...

I took my first yoga class in New York City in 2002. Afterward, I hurried out of the studio, dizzy and sweating, and the first thing I did was call my brother.

"I just did this yoga class," I said. "It was horrible and I nearly fainted. I'm completely sore, and I feel sick," I told him as I sucked on a cigarette. "And I think I love it."

Within 6 weeks, I'd quit smoking, lost 41 lbs, and purchased an unlimited membership. I practiced the next 380 days in a row. The days I couldn't make it to the studio, I practiced at home listening to audios and struggling through sequences in my bedroom.

In a word, I was hooked. I'd gotten the yoga bug, and all these years later, I've never lost it. I'm as crazy about yoga today as I was after that first class, and yoga's ability to transform lives never fails to amaze me.

Today, I'm a yoga teacher, trainer, studio owner, and yoga entrepreneur; but at heart, I'm the same yoga bum I've always been, skipping work to take my favorite classes and cancelling social invitations to get in an extra hour of practice.

For dedicated students, yoga is magic. It transcends the obvious mind-body wellness benefits and becomes a way of life. My hope is that you too get hooked. I'd love for you to develop an obsession with practice, lifelong learning and growth. I'd like nothing more than for yoga to take over your life in the best way possible.

Welcome to the YOGABODY community. We're here to democratize yoga, focus on practice and learning, and bring the best mind-body healing tools to the world.

CONTENTS

PRACTICE LOG	11
BREATHING JOURNAL	113
CLASS NOTES	139
PRACTICE TEACHING	191
YOGABODY STYLE ORIGINS	197
MISC. NOTES	199

Twenty years from now, you will be more disappointed by the things that you didn't do than by the ones you did do, so throw off the bowlines, sail away from safe harbor, and catch the trade winds in your sails.

Explore, Dream, Discover.

— Mark Twain

PRACTICE LOG

Your personal practice is your greatest teacher, always. As part of your training requirement, you need to log 100 classes at approved studios and use this journal to document your journey.

You'll find a wide variety of yoga class styles on offer in most areas, but Ashtanga-Vinyasa based classes are the most-common worldwide, and it's usually very easy to find studios and teachers following this tradition (or some close variation).

Since YOGABODY classes tend to be vinyasa-based, athletic in nature, and vigorous; we recommend you seek out similar classes for your practice. Common styles and class names to look for include: Ashtanga, Vinyasa, Power Yoga or Flow Yoga classes.

Most classes and studios are approved, but if in doubt, check with your teaching mentor.

We also suggest that you take at least 20% of your classes in new and different styles—things you might not normally be interested in. Great teachers are experienced and educated in a variety of approaches to yoga, not close-minded or dogmatic.

If you have a home studio that you love, it's great to focus your training there; but whenever possible, while traveling or in a new city, try to experience new and different teachers and classes. You'll pick up little things along your journey that will greatly add to your teaching voice and your unique teaching style in the future. Never overlook an opportunity to learn.

This Practice Journal has two parts. This first part is simply a long list of all your classes attended with the most basic information. The second part is where you privately review and make notes on some of your class experiences. This is where the real learning happens, but we've positioned it later in the book so you can keep it private. In most cases, it's not appropriate to tell your teachers or studios that you are reviewing their classes—that might make them uncomfortable. This is not for the public, it's just for you, so we recommend you keep your personal notes personal and private as a courtesy to everyone.

NOTE: if you have any questions about the class style you're considering, choices or options, please check in with your teaching mentor. Your teaching mentor is here to help you get the most of your training.

CLASS 01

Date: _____ Duration: _____

Class Name: _____

Studio Name: _____

Teacher Name: _____

Teacher Signature*:

_____
*Please sign to indicate that this student attended your class

CLASS 02

Date: _____ Duration: _____

Class Name: _____

Studio Name: _____

Teacher Name: _____

Teacher Signature*:

_____
*Please sign to indicate that this student attended your class

You miss 100% of the shots you don't take.
— *Wayne Gretzky*

▶◀ CLASS 03 ▶◀

Date: _____ Duration: _____

Class Name: _____

Studio Name: _____

Teacher Name: _____

Teacher Signature*:

_____
*Please sign to indicate that this student attended your class

▶◀ CLASS 04 ▶◀

Date: _____ Duration: _____

Class Name: _____

Studio Name: _____

Teacher Name: _____

Teacher Signature*:

_____
*Please sign to indicate that this student attended your class

Life is 10% what happens to me and 90% of how I react to it.

— *Charles Swindoll*

CLASS 05

Date: _____ Duration: _____

Class Name: _____

Studio Name: _____

Teacher Name: _____

Teacher Signature*:

_____
*Please sign to indicate that this student attended your class

CLASS 06

Date: _____ Duration: _____

Class Name: _____

Studio Name: _____

Teacher Name: _____

Teacher Signature*:

_____
*Please sign to indicate that this student attended your class

*I am not a product of my circumstances.
I am a product of my decisions.*

— *Stephen Covey*

CLASS 07

Date: _____ Duration: _____

Class Name: _____

Studio Name: _____

Teacher Name: _____

Teacher Signature*:

_____
*Please sign to indicate that this student attended your class

CLASS 08

Date: _____ Duration: _____

Class Name: _____

Studio Name: _____

Teacher Name: _____

Teacher Signature*:

_____
*Please sign to indicate that this student attended your class

I've learned that people will forget what you said, people will forget what you did, but people will never forget how you made them feel.

— *Maya Angelou*

CLASS 09

Date: _____ Duration: _____

Class Name: _____

Studio Name: _____

Teacher Name: _____

Teacher Signature*:

_____
*Please sign to indicate that this student attended your class

CLASS 10

Date: _____ Duration: _____

Class Name: _____

Studio Name: _____

Teacher Name: _____

Teacher Signature*:

_____
*Please sign to indicate that this student attended your class

Whether you think you can or you think you can't, you're right.

— *Henry Ford*

CLASS 11

Date: _____ Duration: _____

Class Name: _____

Studio Name: _____

Teacher Name: _____

Teacher Signature*:

_____
*Please sign to indicate that this student attended your class

CLASS 12

Date: _____ Duration: _____

Class Name: _____

Studio Name: _____

Teacher Name: _____

Teacher Signature*:

_____
*Please sign to indicate that this student attended your class

The two most important days in your life are the day you are born and the day you find out why.

— *Mark Twain*

CLASS 13

Date: _____ Duration: _____

Class Name: _____

Studio Name: _____

Teacher Name: _____

Teacher Signature*:

_____
*Please sign to indicate that this student attended your class

CLASS 14

Date: _____ Duration: _____

Class Name: _____

Studio Name: _____

Teacher Name: _____

Teacher Signature*:

_____
*Please sign to indicate that this student attended your class

*Whatever you can do, or dream you can, begin it.
Boldness has genius, power and magic in it.*

— *Johann Wolfgang von Goethe*

CLASS 15

Date: _____ Duration: _____

Class Name: _____

Studio Name: _____

Teacher Name: _____

Teacher Signature*:

Please sign to indicate that this student attended your class

CLASS 16

Date: _____ Duration: _____

Class Name: _____

Studio Name: _____

Teacher Name: _____

Teacher Signature*:

Please sign to indicate that this student attended your class

*People often say that motivation doesn't last.
Well, neither does bathing.
That's why we recommend it daily.
— Zig Ziglar*

CLASS 17

Date: _____ Duration: _____

Class Name: _____

Studio Name: _____

Teacher Name: _____

Teacher Signature*:

_____

*Please sign to indicate that this student attended your class

CLASS 18

Date: _____ Duration: _____

Class Name: _____

Studio Name: _____

Teacher Name: _____

Teacher Signature*:

_____

*Please sign to indicate that this student attended your class

Life shrinks or expands in proportion to one's courage.
— *Anais Nin*

CLASS 19

Date: _____ Duration: _____

Class Name: _____

Studio Name: _____

Teacher Name: _____

Teacher Signature*:

_____
*Please sign to indicate that this student attended your class

CLASS 20

Date: _____ Duration: _____

Class Name: _____

Studio Name: _____

Teacher Name: _____

Teacher Signature*:

_____
*Please sign to indicate that this student attended your class

*There is only one way to avoid criticism:
do nothing, say nothing, and be nothing.*

— *Aristotle*

CLASS 21

Date: _____ Duration: _____

Class Name: _____

Studio Name: _____

Teacher Name: _____

Teacher Signature*:

*Please sign to indicate that this student attended your class

CLASS 22

Date: _____ Duration: _____

Class Name: _____

Studio Name: _____

Teacher Name: _____

Teacher Signature*:

*Please sign to indicate that this student attended your class

Believe you can and you're halfway there.
— *Theodore Roosevelt*

CLASS 23

Date: _____ Duration: _____

Class Name: _____

Studio Name: _____

Teacher Name: _____

Teacher Signature*:

_____
*Please sign to indicate that this student attended your class

CLASS 24

Date: _____ Duration: _____

Class Name: _____

Studio Name: _____

Teacher Name: _____

Teacher Signature*:

_____
*Please sign to indicate that this student attended your class

How wonderful it is that nobody need to wait a single moment before starting to improve the world.

— *Anne Frank*

CLASS 25

Date: _____ Duration: _____

Class Name: _____

Studio Name: _____

Teacher Name: _____

Teacher Signature*:

_____
*Please sign to indicate that this student attended your class

CLASS 26

Date: _____ Duration: _____

Class Name: _____

Studio Name: _____

Teacher Name: _____

Teacher Signature*:

_____
*Please sign to indicate that this student attended your class

Life is not measured by the number of breaths we take, but by the moments that take our breath away.

— *Maya Angelou*

CLASS 27

Date: _____ Duration: _____

Class Name: _____

Studio Name: _____

Teacher Name: _____

Teacher Signature*:

_____
*Please sign to indicate that this student attended your class

CLASS 28

Date: _____ Duration: _____

Class Name: _____

Studio Name: _____

Teacher Name: _____

Teacher Signature*:

_____
*Please sign to indicate that this student attended your class

If you want to lift yourself up, lift up someone else.
— Booker T. Washington

CLASS 29

Date: _____ Duration: _____

Class Name: _____

Studio Name: _____

Teacher Name: _____

Teacher Signature*:

Please sign to indicate that this student attended your class

CLASS 30

Date: _____ Duration: _____

Class Name: _____

Studio Name: _____

Teacher Name: _____

Teacher Signature*:

Please sign to indicate that this student attended your class

I have been impressed with the urgency of doing. Knowing is not enough; we must apply. Being willing is not enough; we must do.

— *Leonardo da Vinci*

CLASS 31

Date: _____ Duration: _____

Class Name: _____

Studio Name: _____

Teacher Name: _____

Teacher Signature*:

_____

*Please sign to indicate that this student attended your class

CLASS 32

Date: _____ Duration: _____

Class Name: _____

Studio Name: _____

Teacher Name: _____

Teacher Signature*:

_____

*Please sign to indicate that this student attended your class

Limitations live only in our minds. But if we use our imaginations, our possibilities become limitless.

— Jamie Paolinetti

CLASS 33

Date: _____ Duration: _____

Class Name: _____

Studio Name: _____

Teacher Name: _____

Teacher Signature*:

_____
*Please sign to indicate that this student attended your class

CLASS 34

Date: _____ Duration: _____

Class Name: _____

Studio Name: _____

Teacher Name: _____

Teacher Signature*:

_____
*Please sign to indicate that this student attended your class

A person who never made a mistake never tried anything new.

— Albert Einstein

▶◀ CLASS 35 ▶◀

Date: _____ Duration: _____

Class Name: _____

Studio Name: _____

Teacher Name: _____

Teacher Signature*:

_____
*Please sign to indicate that this student attended your class

▶◀ CLASS 36 ▶◀

Date: _____ Duration: _____

Class Name: _____

Studio Name: _____

Teacher Name: _____

Teacher Signature*:

_____
*Please sign to indicate that this student attended your class

There are no traffic jams along the extra mile.
— *Roger Staubach*

CLASS 37

Date: _____ Duration: _____

Class Name: _____

Studio Name: _____

Teacher Name: _____

Teacher Signature*:

_____
*Please sign to indicate that this student attended your class

CLASS 38

Date: _____ Duration: _____

Class Name: _____

Studio Name: _____

Teacher Name: _____

Teacher Signature*:

_____
*Please sign to indicate that this student attended your class

Build your own dreams, or someone else will hire you to build theirs.

— *Farrah Gray*

▶ CLASS 39 ◀

Date: _____ Duration: _____

Class Name: _____

Studio Name: _____

Teacher Name: _____

Teacher Signature*:

_____
*Please sign to indicate that this student attended your class

▶ CLASS 40 ◀

Date: _____ Duration: _____

Class Name: _____

Studio Name: _____

Teacher Name: _____

Teacher Signature*:

_____
*Please sign to indicate that this student attended your class

If you look at what you have in life, you'll always have more. If you look at what you don't have in life, you'll never have enough.

— Oprah Winfrey

CLASS 41

Date: _____ Duration: _____

Class Name: _____

Studio Name: _____

Teacher Name: _____

Teacher Signature*:

_____

*Please sign to indicate that this student attended your class

CLASS 42

Date: _____ Duration: _____

Class Name: _____

Studio Name: _____

Teacher Name: _____

Teacher Signature*:

_____

*Please sign to indicate that this student attended your class

Dreaming, after all, is a form of planning.
— *Gloria Steinem*

CLASS 43

Date: _____ Duration: _____

Class Name: _____

Studio Name: _____

Teacher Name: _____

Teacher Signature*:

_____
*Please sign to indicate that this student attended your class

CLASS 44

Date: _____ Duration: _____

Class Name: _____

Studio Name: _____

Teacher Name: _____

Teacher Signature*:

_____
*Please sign to indicate that this student attended your class

When everything seems to be going against you, remember that the airplane takes off against the wind, not with it.

— Henry Ford

CLASS 45

Date: _____ Duration: _____

Class Name: _____

Studio Name: _____

Teacher Name: _____

Teacher Signature*:

*Please sign to indicate that this student attended your class

CLASS 46

Date: _____ Duration: _____

Class Name: _____

Studio Name: _____

Teacher Name: _____

Teacher Signature*:

*Please sign to indicate that this student attended your class

*It's not the years in your life that count.
It's the life in your years.*

— Abraham Lincoln

▶■ CLASS 47 ■◀

Date: _____ Duration: _____

Class Name: _____

Studio Name: _____

Teacher Name: _____

Teacher Signature*:

_____
*Please sign to indicate that this student attended your class

▶■ CLASS 48 ■◀

Date: _____ Duration: _____

Class Name: _____

Studio Name: _____

Teacher Name: _____

Teacher Signature*:

_____
*Please sign to indicate that this student attended your class

The only place where success comes before work is in the dictionary.

— *Vidal Sassoon*

CLASS 49

Date: _____ Duration: _____

Class Name: _____

Studio Name: _____

Teacher Name: _____

Teacher Signature*:

_____
*Please sign to indicate that this student attended your class

CLASS 50

Date: _____ Duration: _____

Class Name: _____

Studio Name: _____

Teacher Name: _____

Teacher Signature*:

_____
*Please sign to indicate that this student attended your class

Take up one idea. Make that one idea your life - think of it, dream of it, live on that idea. Let the brain, muscles, nerves, every part of your body be full of that idea, and just leave every other idea alone. This is the way to success.

— *Swami Vivekananda*

CLASS 51

Date: _____ Duration: _____

Class Name: _____

Studio Name: _____

Teacher Name: _____

Teacher Signature*:

_____
*Please sign to indicate that this student attended your class

CLASS 52

Date: _____ Duration: _____

Class Name: _____

Studio Name: _____

Teacher Name: _____

Teacher Signature*:

_____
*Please sign to indicate that this student attended your class

*Great minds discuss ideas;
average minds discuss events;
small minds discuss people.*

— *Eleanor Roosevelt*

CLASS 53

Date: _____ Duration: _____

Class Name: _____

Studio Name: _____

Teacher Name: _____

Teacher Signature*:

*Please sign to indicate that this student attended your class

CLASS 54

Date: _____ Duration: _____

Class Name: _____

Studio Name: _____

Teacher Name: _____

Teacher Signature*:

*Please sign to indicate that this student attended your class

What seems to us as bitter trials are often blessings in disguise.

— *Oscar Wilde*

CLASS 55

Date: _____ Duration: _____

Class Name: _____

Studio Name: _____

Teacher Name: _____

Teacher Signature*:

_____
*Please sign to indicate that this student attended your class

CLASS 56

Date: _____ Duration: _____

Class Name: _____

Studio Name: _____

Teacher Name: _____

Teacher Signature*:

_____
*Please sign to indicate that this student attended your class

If you can't explain it simply, you don't understand it well enough.

— *Albert Einstein*

CLASS 57

Date: _____ Duration: _____

Class Name: _____

Studio Name: _____

Teacher Name: _____

Teacher Signature*:

_____
*Please sign to indicate that this student attended your class

CLASS 58

Date: _____ Duration: _____

Class Name: _____

Studio Name: _____

Teacher Name: _____

Teacher Signature*:

_____
*Please sign to indicate that this student attended your class

There are two types of people who will tell you that you cannot make a difference in this world: those who are afraid to try and those who are afraid you will succeed.

— *Ray Goforth*

CLASS 59

Date: _____ Duration: _____

Class Name: _____

Studio Name: _____

Teacher Name: _____

Teacher Signature*:

_____
*Please sign to indicate that this student attended your class

CLASS 60

Date: _____ Duration: _____

Class Name: _____

Studio Name: _____

Teacher Name: _____

Teacher Signature*:

_____
*Please sign to indicate that this student attended your class

No one can make you feel inferior without your consent.
— Eleanor Roosevelt

▶ CLASS 61 ◀

Date: _____ Duration: _____

Class Name: _____

Studio Name: _____

Teacher Name: _____

Teacher Signature*:

_____
*Please sign to indicate that this student attended your class

▶ CLASS 62 ◀

Date: _____ Duration: _____

Class Name: _____

Studio Name: _____

Teacher Name: _____

Teacher Signature*:

_____
*Please sign to indicate that this student attended your class

I find that the harder I work, the more luck I seem to have.

— *Thomas Jefferson*

CLASS 63

Date: _____ Duration: _____

Class Name: _____

Studio Name: _____

Teacher Name: _____

Teacher Signature*:

*Please sign to indicate that this student attended your class

CLASS 64

Date: _____ Duration: _____

Class Name: _____

Studio Name: _____

Teacher Name: _____

Teacher Signature*:

*Please sign to indicate that this student attended your class

Success is the sum of small efforts, repeated day-in and day-out.

— *Robert Collier*

CLASS 65

Date: _____ Duration: _____

Class Name: _____

Studio Name: _____

Teacher Name: _____

Teacher Signature*:

_____
*Please sign to indicate that this student attended your class

CLASS 66

Date: _____ Duration: _____

Class Name: _____

Studio Name: _____

Teacher Name: _____

Teacher Signature*:

_____
*Please sign to indicate that this student attended your class

Two roads diverged in a wood, and I—
I took the one less traveled by,
And that has made all the difference.

— Robert Frost

▶◣ CLASS 67 ◢◀

Date: _____ Duration: _____

Class Name: _____

Studio Name: _____

Teacher Name: _____

Teacher Signature*:

*Please sign to indicate that this student attended your class

▶◣ CLASS 68 ◢◀

Date: _____ Duration: _____

Class Name: _____

Studio Name: _____

Teacher Name: _____

Teacher Signature*:

*Please sign to indicate that this student attended your class

If you always put limits on everything you do, physical or anything else, it will spread into your work and into your life. There are no limits. There are only plateaus, and you must not stay there, you must go beyond them.

— *Bruce Lee*

CLASS 69

Date: _____ Duration: _____

Class Name: _____

Studio Name: _____

Teacher Name: _____

Teacher Signature*:

_____
*Please sign to indicate that this student attended your class

CLASS 70

Date: _____ Duration: _____

Class Name: _____

Studio Name: _____

Teacher Name: _____

Teacher Signature*:

_____
*Please sign to indicate that this student attended your class

The most difficult thing is the decision to act, the rest is merely tenacity.

— *Amelia Earhart*

CLASS 71

Date: _____ Duration: _____

Class Name: _____

Studio Name: _____

Teacher Name: _____

Teacher Signature*:

Please sign to indicate that this student attended your class

CLASS 72

Date: _____ Duration: _____

Class Name: _____

Studio Name: _____

Teacher Name: _____

Teacher Signature*:

Please sign to indicate that this student attended your class

Life isn't about getting and having, it's about giving and being.

— *Kevin Kruse*

CLASS 73

Date: _____ Duration: _____

Class Name: _____

Studio Name: _____

Teacher Name: _____

Teacher Signature*:

_____
*Please sign to indicate that this student attended your class

CLASS 74

Date: _____ Duration: _____

Class Name: _____

Studio Name: _____

Teacher Name: _____

Teacher Signature*:

_____
*Please sign to indicate that this student attended your class

The best time to plant a tree was 20 years ago. The second best time is now.

— *Chinese Proverb*

▶— CLASS 75 —◀

Date: _____ Duration: _____

Class Name: _____

Studio Name: _____

Teacher Name: _____

Teacher Signature*:

*Please sign to indicate that this student attended your class

▶— CLASS 76 —◀

Date: _____ Duration: _____

Class Name: _____

Studio Name: _____

Teacher Name: _____

Teacher Signature*:

*Please sign to indicate that this student attended your class

When I stand before God at the end of my life, I would hope that I would not have a single bit of talent left and could say, I used everything you gave me.

— *Erma Bombeck*

CLASS 77

Date: _____ Duration: _____

Class Name: _____

Studio Name: _____

Teacher Name: _____

Teacher Signature*:

*Please sign to indicate that this student attended your class

CLASS 78

Date: _____ Duration: _____

Class Name: _____

Studio Name: _____

Teacher Name: _____

Teacher Signature*:

*Please sign to indicate that this student attended your class

Everything you've ever wanted is on the other side of fear.

— *George Addair*

CLASS 79

Date: _____ Duration: _____

Class Name: _____

Studio Name: _____

Teacher Name: _____

Teacher Signature*:

_____
*Please sign to indicate that this student attended your class

CLASS 80

Date: _____ Duration: _____

Class Name: _____

Studio Name: _____

Teacher Name: _____

Teacher Signature*:

_____
*Please sign to indicate that this student attended your class

*No matter what people tell you,
words and ideas can change the world.*
— *Robin Williams*

CLASS 81

Date: _____ Duration: _____

Class Name: _____

Studio Name: _____

Teacher Name: _____

Teacher Signature*:

*Please sign to indicate that this student attended your class

CLASS 82

Date: _____ Duration: _____

Class Name: _____

Studio Name: _____

Teacher Name: _____

Teacher Signature*:

*Please sign to indicate that this student attended your class

When I let go of what I am, I become what I might be.
  — *Lao Tzu*

CLASS 83

Date: _____ Duration: _____

Class Name: _____

Studio Name: _____

Teacher Name: _____

Teacher Signature*:

_____
*Please sign to indicate that this student attended your class

CLASS 84

Date: _____ Duration: _____

Class Name: _____

Studio Name: _____

Teacher Name: _____

Teacher Signature*:

_____
*Please sign to indicate that this student attended your class

Too many of us are not living our dreams because we are living our fears.

— *Les Brown*

CLASS 85

Date: _____ Duration: _____

Class Name: _____

Studio Name: _____

Teacher Name: _____

Teacher Signature*:

_____
*Please sign to indicate that this student attended your class

CLASS 86

Date: _____ Duration: _____

Class Name: _____

Studio Name: _____

Teacher Name: _____

Teacher Signature*:

_____
*Please sign to indicate that this student attended your class

It is never too late to be what you might have been.
— *George Eliot*

CLASS 87

Date: _____ Duration: _____

Class Name: _____

Studio Name: _____

Teacher Name: _____

Teacher Signature*:

*Please sign to indicate that this student attended your class

CLASS 88

Date: _____ Duration: _____

Class Name: _____

Studio Name: _____

Teacher Name: _____

Teacher Signature*:

*Please sign to indicate that this student attended your class

Dream big and dare to fail.
— *Norman Vaughan*

CLASS 89

Date: _____ Duration: _____

Class Name: _____

Studio Name: _____

Teacher Name: _____

Teacher Signature*:

Please sign to indicate that this student attended your class

CLASS 90

Date: _____ Duration: _____

Class Name: _____

Studio Name: _____

Teacher Name: _____

Teacher Signature*:

Please sign to indicate that this student attended your class

Nothing is impossible, the word itself says, "I'm possible!"

— Audrey Hepburn

CLASS 91

Date: _____ Duration: _____

Class Name: _____

Studio Name: _____

Teacher Name: _____

Teacher Signature*:

_____
*Please sign to indicate that this student attended your class

CLASS 92

Date: _____ Duration: _____

Class Name: _____

Studio Name: _____

Teacher Name: _____

Teacher Signature*:

_____
*Please sign to indicate that this student attended your class

Life is what we make it, always has been, always will be.

— *Grandma Moses*

CLASS 93

Date: _____ Duration: _____

Class Name: _____

Studio Name: _____

Teacher Name: _____

Teacher Signature*:

_____
*Please sign to indicate that this student attended your class

CLASS 94

Date: _____ Duration: _____

Class Name: _____

Studio Name: _____

Teacher Name: _____

Teacher Signature*:

_____
*Please sign to indicate that this student attended your class

Start by doing what's necessary; then do what's possible; and suddenly you are doing the impossible.

— *Francis of Assisi*

► CLASS 95 ◄

Date: _____ Duration: _____

Class Name: _____

Studio Name: _____

Teacher Name: _____

Teacher Signature*:

*Please sign to indicate that this student attended your class

► CLASS 96 ◄

Date: _____ Duration: _____

Class Name: _____

Studio Name: _____

Teacher Name: _____

Teacher Signature*:

*Please sign to indicate that this student attended your class

We know what we are, but know not what we may be.
— *William Shakespeare*

CLASS 97

Date: _____ Duration: _____

Class Name: _____

Studio Name: _____

Teacher Name: _____

Teacher Signature*:

*Please sign to indicate that this student attended your class

CLASS 98

Date: _____ Duration: _____

Class Name: _____

Studio Name: _____

Teacher Name: _____

Teacher Signature*:

*Please sign to indicate that this student attended your class

No act of kindness, no matter how small, is ever wasted.
　　　　　　　　　　　— Aesop

CLASS 99

Date: _____ Duration: _____

Class Name: _____

Studio Name: _____

Teacher Name: _____

Teacher Signature*:

_____
*Please sign to indicate that this student attended your class

CLASS 100

Date: _____ Duration: _____

Class Name: _____

Studio Name: _____

Teacher Name: _____

Teacher Signature*:

_____
*Please sign to indicate that this student attended your class

To laugh often and much; to win the respect of intelligent people and the affection of children... to leave the world a better place... to know even one life has breathed easier because you have lived. This is to have succeeded.

— Ralph Waldo Emerson

BREATHING JOURNAL

Breathing is one of the most powerful yoga tools for shifting mood, relieving stress, and taking control over our central nervous system. During this course, you'll learn a number of different breathing techniques, and as part of your training, you're required to log a minimum of 25 at-home practice sessions (self-guided).

During your teaching assessment, you'll need to lead your teaching mentor through all the practices learned, so the more you practice, the more confident you'll be to teach.

For visual reference and detailed instruction, please refer to your online modules on breathing.

🌬 BREATHING SESSION 01 🌬

Date: _____   Duration: _____

Time of Day: ☐ morning   ☐ afternoon
               ☐ evening   ☐ before bed

Technique/s Practiced: _____

How do you Feel?   ☐ balanced   ☐ anxious   ☐ frustrated
                   ☐ tired   ☐ energized   ☐ not sure

Notes/Observations?

🌬 BREATHING SESSION 02 🌬

Date: _____   Duration: _____

Time of Day: ☐ morning   ☐ afternoon
               ☐ evening   ☐ before bed

Technique/s Practiced: _____

How do you Feel?   ☐ balanced   ☐ anxious   ☐ frustrated
                   ☐ tired   ☐ energized   ☐ not sure

Notes/Observations?

🌬 BREATHING SESSION 03 🌬

Date: _____ Duration: _____

Time of Day: ☐ morning   ☐ afternoon
              ☐ evening   ☐ before bed

Technique/s Practiced: _____

How do you Feel? ☐ balanced ☐ anxious   ☐ frustrated
                  ☐ tired   ☐ energized ☐ not sure

Notes/Observations?

🌬 BREATHING SESSION 04 🌬

Date: _____ Duration: _____

Time of Day: ☐ morning   ☐ afternoon
              ☐ evening   ☐ before bed

Technique/s Practiced: _____

How do you Feel? ☐ balanced ☐ anxious   ☐ frustrated
                  ☐ tired   ☐ energized ☐ not sure

Notes/Observations?

BREATHING SESSION 05

Date: _____ Duration: _____

Time of Day: ☐ morning   ☐ afternoon
              ☐ evening   ☐ before bed

Technique/s Practiced: _____

How do you Feel? ☐ balanced   ☐ anxious   ☐ frustrated
                  ☐ tired   ☐ energized ☐ not sure

Notes/Observations?

BREATHING SESSION 06

Date: _____ Duration: _____

Time of Day: ☐ morning   ☐ afternoon
              ☐ evening   ☐ before bed

Technique/s Practiced: _____

How do you Feel? ☐ balanced   ☐ anxious   ☐ frustrated
                  ☐ tired   ☐ energized ☐ not sure

Notes/Observations?

BREATHING SESSION 07

Date: _____ Duration: _____

Time of Day: ☐ morning   ☐ afternoon
              ☐ evening   ☐ before bed

Technique/s Practiced: _____

How do you Feel? ☐ balanced   ☐ anxious   ☐ frustrated
                  ☐ tired   ☐ energized ☐ not sure

Notes/Observations?

BREATHING SESSION 08

Date: _____ Duration: _____

Time of Day: ☐ morning   ☐ afternoon
              ☐ evening   ☐ before bed

Technique/s Practiced: _____

How do you Feel? ☐ balanced   ☐ anxious   ☐ frustrated
                  ☐ tired   ☐ energized ☐ not sure

Notes/Observations?

☴ BREATHING SESSION 09 ☴

Date: _____   Duration: _____

Time of Day: ☐ morning   ☐ afternoon
               ☐ evening   ☐ before bed

Technique/s Practiced: _____

How do you Feel?   ☐ balanced   ☐ anxious   ☐ frustrated
                   ☐ tired   ☐ energized   ☐ not sure

Notes/Observations?

☴ BREATHING SESSION 10 ☴

Date: _____   Duration: _____

Time of Day: ☐ morning   ☐ afternoon
               ☐ evening   ☐ before bed

Technique/s Practiced: _____

How do you Feel?   ☐ balanced   ☐ anxious   ☐ frustrated
                   ☐ tired   ☐ energized   ☐ not sure

Notes/Observations?

BREATHING SESSION 11

Date: _____ Duration: _____

Time of Day: ☐ morning   ☐ afternoon
             ☐ evening   ☐ before bed

Technique/s Practiced: _____

How do you Feel? ☐ balanced ☐ anxious   ☐ frustrated
                  ☐ tired   ☐ energized ☐ not sure

Notes/Observations?

BREATHING SESSION 12

Date: _____ Duration: _____

Time of Day: ☐ morning   ☐ afternoon
             ☐ evening   ☐ before bed

Technique/s Practiced: _____

How do you Feel? ☐ balanced ☐ anxious   ☐ frustrated
                  ☐ tired   ☐ energized ☐ not sure

Notes/Observations?

BREATHING SESSION 13

Date: _____ Duration: _____

Time of Day: ☐ morning   ☐ afternoon
              ☐ evening   ☐ before bed

Technique/s Practiced: _____

How do you Feel? ☐ balanced   ☐ anxious   ☐ frustrated
                  ☐ tired   ☐ energized ☐ not sure

Notes/Observations?

BREATHING SESSION 14

Date: _____ Duration: _____

Time of Day: ☐ morning   ☐ afternoon
              ☐ evening   ☐ before bed

Technique/s Practiced: _____

How do you Feel? ☐ balanced   ☐ anxious   ☐ frustrated
                  ☐ tired   ☐ energized ☐ not sure

Notes/Observations?

BREATHING SESSION 15

Date: _____ Duration: _____

Time of Day: ☐ morning ☐ afternoon
☐ evening ☐ before bed

Technique/s Practiced: _____

How do you Feel? ☐ balanced ☐ anxious ☐ frustrated
☐ tired ☐ energized ☐ not sure

Notes/Observations?

BREATHING SESSION 16

Date: _____ Duration: _____

Time of Day: ☐ morning ☐ afternoon
☐ evening ☐ before bed

Technique/s Practiced: _____

How do you Feel? ☐ balanced ☐ anxious ☐ frustrated
☐ tired ☐ energized ☐ not sure

Notes/Observations?

🌬 BREATHING SESSION 17 🌬

Date: _____ Duration: _____

Time of Day: ☐ morning   ☐ afternoon
              ☐ evening   ☐ before bed

Technique/s Practiced: _____

How do you Feel? ☐ balanced ☐ anxious   ☐ frustrated
                  ☐ tired   ☐ energized ☐ not sure

Notes/Observations?

🌬 BREATHING SESSION 18 🌬

Date: _____ Duration: _____

Time of Day: ☐ morning   ☐ afternoon
              ☐ evening   ☐ before bed

Technique/s Practiced: _____

How do you Feel? ☐ balanced ☐ anxious   ☐ frustrated
                  ☐ tired   ☐ energized ☐ not sure

Notes/Observations?

BREATHING SESSION 19

Date: _____ Duration: _____

Time of Day: ☐ morning   ☐ afternoon
              ☐ evening   ☐ before bed

Technique/s Practiced: _____

How do you Feel? ☐ balanced ☐ anxious   ☐ frustrated
                  ☐ tired   ☐ energized ☐ not sure

Notes/Observations?

BREATHING SESSION 20

Date: _____ Duration: _____

Time of Day: ☐ morning   ☐ afternoon
              ☐ evening   ☐ before bed

Technique/s Practiced: _____

How do you Feel? ☐ balanced ☐ anxious   ☐ frustrated
                  ☐ tired   ☐ energized ☐ not sure

Notes/Observations?

༄ BREATHING SESSION 21

Date: _____ Duration: _____

Time of Day: ☐ morning   ☐ afternoon
              ☐ evening   ☐ before bed

Technique/s Practiced: _____

How do you Feel? ☐ balanced ☐ anxious   ☐ frustrated
                  ☐ tired   ☐ energized ☐ not sure

Notes/Observations?

༄ BREATHING SESSION 22

Date: _____ Duration: _____

Time of Day: ☐ morning   ☐ afternoon
              ☐ evening   ☐ before bed

Technique/s Practiced: _____

How do you Feel? ☐ balanced ☐ anxious   ☐ frustrated
                  ☐ tired   ☐ energized ☐ not sure

Notes/Observations?

BREATHING SESSION 23

Date: _____ Duration: _____

Time of Day: ☐ morning   ☐ afternoon
              ☐ evening   ☐ before bed

Technique/s Practiced: _____

How do you Feel? ☐ balanced ☐ anxious   ☐ frustrated
                  ☐ tired   ☐ energized ☐ not sure

Notes/Observations?

BREATHING SESSION 24

Date: _____ Duration: _____

Time of Day: ☐ morning   ☐ afternoon
              ☐ evening   ☐ before bed

Technique/s Practiced: _____

How do you Feel? ☐ balanced ☐ anxious   ☐ frustrated
                  ☐ tired   ☐ energized ☐ not sure

Notes/Observations?

🌬 BREATHING SESSION 25 🌬

Date: _____ Duration: _____

Time of Day: ☐ morning   ☐ afternoon
              ☐ evening   ☐ before bed

Technique/s Practiced: _____

How do you Feel? ☐ balanced   ☐ anxious   ☐ frustrated
                  ☐ tired   ☐ energized ☐ not sure

Notes/Observations?

🌬 BREATHING SESSION 26 🌬

Date: _____ Duration: _____

Time of Day: ☐ morning   ☐ afternoon
              ☐ evening   ☐ before bed

Technique/s Practiced: _____

How do you Feel? ☐ balanced   ☐ anxious   ☐ frustrated
                  ☐ tired   ☐ energized ☐ not sure

Notes/Observations?

BREATHING SESSION 27

Date: _____ Duration: _____

Time of Day: ☐ morning   ☐ afternoon
              ☐ evening   ☐ before bed

Technique/s Practiced: _____

How do you Feel? ☐ balanced ☐ anxious   ☐ frustrated
                  ☐ tired   ☐ energized ☐ not sure

Notes/Observations?

BREATHING SESSION 28

Date: _____ Duration: _____

Time of Day: ☐ morning   ☐ afternoon
              ☐ evening   ☐ before bed

Technique/s Practiced: _____

How do you Feel? ☐ balanced ☐ anxious   ☐ frustrated
                  ☐ tired   ☐ energized ☐ not sure

Notes/Observations?

🌬 BREATHING SESSION 29 🌬

Date: _____ Duration: _____

Time of Day: ☐ morning   ☐ afternoon
              ☐ evening   ☐ before bed

Technique/s Practiced: _____

How do you Feel? ☐ balanced   ☐ anxious   ☐ frustrated
                  ☐ tired   ☐ energized ☐ not sure

Notes/Observations?

🌬 BREATHING SESSION 30 🌬

Date: _____ Duration: _____

Time of Day: ☐ morning   ☐ afternoon
              ☐ evening   ☐ before bed

Technique/s Practiced: _____

How do you Feel? ☐ balanced   ☐ anxious   ☐ frustrated
                  ☐ tired   ☐ energized ☐ not sure

Notes/Observations?

BREATHING SESSION 31

Date: _____ Duration: _____

Time of Day: ☐ morning   ☐ afternoon
              ☐ evening   ☐ before bed

Technique/s Practiced: _____

How do you Feel? ☐ balanced ☐ anxious   ☐ frustrated
                  ☐ tired   ☐ energized ☐ not sure

Notes/Observations?

BREATHING SESSION 32

Date: _____ Duration: _____

Time of Day: ☐ morning   ☐ afternoon
              ☐ evening   ☐ before bed

Technique/s Practiced: _____

How do you Feel? ☐ balanced ☐ anxious   ☐ frustrated
                  ☐ tired   ☐ energized ☐ not sure

Notes/Observations?

BREATHING SESSION 33

Date: _____ Duration: _____

Time of Day: ☐ morning   ☐ afternoon
               ☐ evening   ☐ before bed

Technique/s Practiced: _____

How do you Feel?   ☐ balanced   ☐ anxious   ☐ frustrated
                   ☐ tired   ☐ energized ☐ not sure

Notes/Observations?

BREATHING SESSION 34

Date: _____ Duration: _____

Time of Day: ☐ morning   ☐ afternoon
               ☐ evening   ☐ before bed

Technique/s Practiced: _____

How do you Feel?   ☐ balanced   ☐ anxious   ☐ frustrated
                   ☐ tired   ☐ energized ☐ not sure

Notes/Observations?

BREATHING SESSION 35

Date: _____ Duration: _____

Time of Day: ☐ morning   ☐ afternoon
              ☐ evening   ☐ before bed

Technique/s Practiced: _____

How do you Feel? ☐ balanced ☐ anxious   ☐ frustrated
                  ☐ tired   ☐ energized ☐ not sure

Notes/Observations?

BREATHING SESSION 36

Date: _____ Duration: _____

Time of Day: ☐ morning   ☐ afternoon
              ☐ evening   ☐ before bed

Technique/s Practiced: _____

How do you Feel? ☐ balanced ☐ anxious   ☐ frustrated
                  ☐ tired   ☐ energized ☐ not sure

Notes/Observations?

➰ BREATHING SESSION 37 ➰

Date: _____ Duration: _____

Time of Day: ☐ morning ☐ afternoon
              ☐ evening ☐ before bed

Technique/s Practiced: _____

How do you Feel? ☐ balanced ☐ anxious   ☐ frustrated
                  ☐ tired   ☐ energized ☐ not sure

Notes/Observations?

➰ BREATHING SESSION 38 ➰

Date: _____ Duration: _____

Time of Day: ☐ morning ☐ afternoon
              ☐ evening ☐ before bed

Technique/s Practiced: _____

How do you Feel? ☐ balanced ☐ anxious   ☐ frustrated
                  ☐ tired   ☐ energized ☐ not sure

Notes/Observations?

BREATHING SESSION 39

Date: _____ Duration: _____

Time of Day: ☐ morning   ☐ afternoon
              ☐ evening   ☐ before bed

Technique/s Practiced: _____

How do you Feel? ☐ balanced ☐ anxious   ☐ frustrated
                  ☐ tired   ☐ energized ☐ not sure

Notes/Observations?

BREATHING SESSION 40

Date: _____ Duration: _____

Time of Day: ☐ morning   ☐ afternoon
              ☐ evening   ☐ before bed

Technique/s Practiced: _____

How do you Feel? ☐ balanced ☐ anxious   ☐ frustrated
                  ☐ tired   ☐ energized ☐ not sure

Notes/Observations?

BREATHING SESSION 41

Date: _____ Duration: _____

Time of Day: ☐ morning   ☐ afternoon
              ☐ evening   ☐ before bed

Technique/s Practiced: _____

How do you Feel? ☐ balanced   ☐ anxious   ☐ frustrated
                  ☐ tired   ☐ energized   ☐ not sure

Notes/Observations?

BREATHING SESSION 42

Date: _____ Duration: _____

Time of Day: ☐ morning   ☐ afternoon
              ☐ evening   ☐ before bed

Technique/s Practiced: _____

How do you Feel? ☐ balanced   ☐ anxious   ☐ frustrated
                  ☐ tired   ☐ energized   ☐ not sure

Notes/Observations?

BREATHING SESSION 43

Date: _____ Duration: _____

Time of Day: ☐ morning   ☐ afternoon
              ☐ evening   ☐ before bed

Technique/s Practiced: _____

How do you Feel? ☐ balanced   ☐ anxious   ☐ frustrated
                  ☐ tired   ☐ energized ☐ not sure

Notes/Observations?

BREATHING SESSION 44

Date: _____ Duration: _____

Time of Day: ☐ morning   ☐ afternoon
              ☐ evening   ☐ before bed

Technique/s Practiced: _____

How do you Feel? ☐ balanced   ☐ anxious   ☐ frustrated
                  ☐ tired   ☐ energized ☐ not sure

Notes/Observations?

🌬 BREATHING SESSION 45 🌬

Date: _____ Duration: _____

Time of Day: ☐ morning   ☐ afternoon
              ☐ evening   ☐ before bed

Technique/s Practiced: _____

How do you Feel? ☐ balanced ☐ anxious   ☐ frustrated
                  ☐ tired   ☐ energized ☐ not sure

Notes/Observations?

🌬 BREATHING SESSION 46 🌬

Date: _____ Duration: _____

Time of Day: ☐ morning   ☐ afternoon
              ☐ evening   ☐ before bed

Technique/s Practiced: _____

How do you Feel? ☐ balanced ☐ anxious   ☐ frustrated
                  ☐ tired   ☐ energized ☐ not sure

Notes/Observations?

BREATHING SESSION 47

Date: _____   Duration: _____

Time of Day: ☐ morning   ☐ afternoon
              ☐ evening   ☐ before bed

Technique/s Practiced: _____

How do you Feel? ☐ balanced   ☐ anxious   ☐ frustrated
                  ☐ tired   ☐ energized ☐ not sure

Notes/Observations?

BREATHING SESSION 48

Date: _____   Duration: _____

Time of Day: ☐ morning   ☐ afternoon
              ☐ evening   ☐ before bed

Technique/s Practiced: _____

How do you Feel? ☐ balanced   ☐ anxious   ☐ frustrated
                  ☐ tired   ☐ energized ☐ not sure

Notes/Observations?

🌬 BREATHING SESSION 49 🌬

Date: _____ Duration: _____

Time of Day: ☐ morning   ☐ afternoon
              ☐ evening   ☐ before bed

Technique/s Practiced: _____

How do you Feel? ☐ balanced   ☐ anxious   ☐ frustrated
                  ☐ tired   ☐ energized ☐ not sure

Notes/Observations?

🌬 BREATHING SESSION 50 🌬

Date: _____ Duration: _____

Time of Day: ☐ morning   ☐ afternoon
              ☐ evening   ☐ before bed

Technique/s Practiced: _____

How do you Feel? ☐ balanced   ☐ anxious   ☐ frustrated
                  ☐ tired   ☐ energized ☐ not sure

Notes/Observations?

OBSERVATIONS, CLASS NOTES, & LEARNING

As an aspiring teacher, each and every class you take is a learning opportunity, but in order to get the most of each class, you need to document what you've experienced. This is "for your eyes only" and is not meant to be shared with your teachers or any other students—that would not be appropriate.

When reviewing each class, try to be thoughtful, thorough, and view the class as taught by a soon-to-be colleague. What did you love? What would you do differently? What worked? What was clumsy?

The simple practice of keeping diligent class notes will increase your awareness about what makes a great class and will help you to model that in your teaching.

It's suggested that you take your class notes the same day you take your class, so it's still fresh in your memory. We do not recommend you do this at the studio or in front of any other students or studio staff members as that might make them feel uncomfortable.

Remember, these notes are private. They are for you and your learning—not to criticize or give unsolicited feedback to others.

As a student, your practice and experiences are constantly changing. As you begin to teach, your experiences change even more, and it's very important you make note of what works, what doesn't work, what you like and dislike about the various classes you've taken.

As teachers, we are nothing more than the sum of our experiences, and the more you document and record your actual experiences—the more you'll learn.

100 yoga classes is not a big number, but when you record your experiences in this fashion, it's enough to attain professional-level proficiency as a teacher.

CLASS 01 NOTES

Teacher/Studio _____

Class Name: _____ Date of Attendance: _____

Voice Projection:

☐ always clear / easy to hear
☐ mostly clear / easy to hear
☐ some instructions were lost, unclear or confusing
☐ many things were lost (not able to hear)

Physical Assists / Adjustments?

☐ lots of adjustments throughout class
☐ good number of adjustments
☐ some adjustments
☐ lacking adjustments

Energy?

☐ great energy throughout class
☐ good energy
☐ some ups and downs
☐ lacking energy

Rhythm & Pacing?

☐ great pacing, great timing
☐ good pacing & timing
☐ too fast or too slow at times
☐ rhythm felt off

Connection with Students?

- ☐ great connection, used students' names, held group together
- ☐ good connection
- ☐ some students connected, others a little lost
- ☐ felt disconnected

Organization / Planning?

- ☐ teacher available before/after class to chat with students?
- ☐ started/finished on time?
- ☐ was the music appropriate volume and choice?
- ☐ was the mat arrangement / room arrangement appropriate?
- ☐ was the temperature of the room appropriate?

Best thing about the class?

Any areas that felt a little off today?

Other Comments?

CLASS 02 NOTES

Teacher/Studio _____

Class Name: _____ Date of Attendance: _____

Voice Projection:

☐ always clear / easy to hear
☐ mostly clear / easy to hear
☐ some instructions were lost, unclear or confusing
☐ many things were lost (not able to hear)

Physical Assists / Adjustments?

☐ lots of adjustments throughout class
☐ good number of adjustments
☐ some adjustments
☐ lacking adjustments

Energy?

☐ great energy throughout class
☐ good energy
☐ some ups and downs
☐ lacking energy

Rhythm & Pacing?

☐ great pacing, great timing
☐ good pacing & timing
☐ too fast or too slow at times
☐ rhythm felt off

Connection with Students?

- ☐ great connection, used students' names, held group together
- ☐ good connection
- ☐ some students connected, others a little lost
- ☐ felt disconnected

Organization / Planning?

- ☐ teacher available before/after class to chat with students?
- ☐ started/finished on time?
- ☐ was the music appropriate volume and choice?
- ☐ was the mat arrangement / room arrangement appropriate?
- ☐ was the temperature of the room appropriate?

Best thing about the class?

Any areas that felt a little off today?

Other Comments?

◤ CLASS 03 NOTES ◥

Teacher/Studio _____

Class Name: _____ Date of Attendance: _____

Voice Projection:

☐ always clear / easy to hear
☐ mostly clear / easy to hear
☐ some instructions were lost, unclear or confusing
☐ many things were lost (not able to hear)

Physical Assists / Adjustments?

☐ lots of adjustments throughout class
☐ good number of adjustments
☐ some adjustments
☐ lacking adjustments

Energy?

☐ great energy throughout class
☐ good energy
☐ some ups and downs
☐ lacking energy

Rhythm & Pacing?

☐ great pacing, great timing
☐ good pacing & timing
☐ too fast or too slow at times
☐ rhythm felt off

Connection with Students?

- ☐ great connection, used students' names, held group together
- ☐ good connection
- ☐ some students connected, others a little lost
- ☐ felt disconnected

Organization / Planning?

- ☐ teacher available before/after class to chat with students?
- ☐ started/finished on time?
- ☐ was the music appropriate volume and choice?
- ☐ was the mat arrangement / room arrangement appropriate?
- ☐ was the temperature of the room appropriate?

Best thing about the class?

Any areas that felt a little off today?

Other Comments?

CLASS 04 NOTES

Teacher/Studio _____

Class Name: _____ Date of Attendance: _____

Voice Projection:

☐ always clear / easy to hear
☐ mostly clear / easy to hear
☐ some instructions were lost, unclear or confusing
☐ many things were lost (not able to hear)

Physical Assists / Adjustments?

☐ lots of adjustments throughout class
☐ good number of adjustments
☐ some adjustments
☐ lacking adjustments

Energy?

☐ great energy throughout class
☐ good energy
☐ some ups and downs
☐ lacking energy

Rhythm & Pacing?

☐ great pacing, great timing
☐ good pacing & timing
☐ too fast or too slow at times
☐ rhythm felt off

Connection with Students?

- ☐ great connection, used students' names, held group together
- ☐ good connection
- ☐ some students connected, others a little lost
- ☐ felt disconnected

Organization / Planning?

- ☐ teacher available before/after class to chat with students?
- ☐ started/finished on time?
- ☐ was the music appropriate volume and choice?
- ☐ was the mat arrangement / room arrangement appropriate?
- ☐ was the temperature of the room appropriate?

Best thing about the class?

Any areas that felt a little off today?

Other Comments?

CLASS 05 NOTES

Teacher/Studio _____

Class Name: _____ Date of Attendance: _____

Voice Projection:

☐ always clear / easy to hear
☐ mostly clear / easy to hear
☐ some instructions were lost, unclear or confusing
☐ many things were lost (not able to hear)

Physical Assists / Adjustments?

☐ lots of adjustments throughout class
☐ good number of adjustments
☐ some adjustments
☐ lacking adjustments

Energy?

☐ great energy throughout class
☐ good energy
☐ some ups and downs
☐ lacking energy

Rhythm & Pacing?

☐ great pacing, great timing
☐ good pacing & timing
☐ too fast or too slow at times
☐ rhythm felt off

Connection with Students?

- ☐ great connection, used students' names, held group together
- ☐ good connection
- ☐ some students connected, others a little lost
- ☐ felt disconnected

Organization / Planning?

- ☐ teacher available before/after class to chat with students?
- ☐ started/finished on time?
- ☐ was the music appropriate volume and choice?
- ☐ was the mat arrangement / room arrangement appropriate?
- ☐ was the temperature of the room appropriate?

Best thing about the class?

Any areas that felt a little off today?

Other Comments?

CLASS 06 NOTES

Teacher/Studio _____

Class Name: _____ Date of Attendance: _____

Voice Projection:

☐ always clear / easy to hear
☐ mostly clear / easy to hear
☐ some instructions were lost, unclear or confusing
☐ many things were lost (not able to hear)

Physical Assists / Adjustments?

☐ lots of adjustments throughout class
☐ good number of adjustments
☐ some adjustments
☐ lacking adjustments

Energy?

☐ great energy throughout class
☐ good energy
☐ some ups and downs
☐ lacking energy

Rhythm & Pacing?

☐ great pacing, great timing
☐ good pacing & timing
☐ too fast or too slow at times
☐ rhythm felt off

Connection with Students?

- ☐ great connection, used students' names, held group together
- ☐ good connection
- ☐ some students connected, others a little lost
- ☐ felt disconnected

Organization / Planning?

- ☐ teacher available before/after class to chat with students?
- ☐ started/finished on time?
- ☐ was the music appropriate volume and choice?
- ☐ was the mat arrangement / room arrangement appropriate?
- ☐ was the temperature of the room appropriate?

Best thing about the class?

Any areas that felt a little off today?

Other Comments?

CLASS 07 NOTES

Teacher/Studio _____

Class Name: _____ Date of Attendance: _____

Voice Projection:

☐ always clear / easy to hear
☐ mostly clear / easy to hear
☐ some instructions were lost, unclear or confusing
☐ many things were lost (not able to hear)

Physical Assists / Adjustments?

☐ lots of adjustments throughout class
☐ good number of adjustments
☐ some adjustments
☐ lacking adjustments

Energy?

☐ great energy throughout class
☐ good energy
☐ some ups and downs
☐ lacking energy

Rhythm & Pacing?

☐ great pacing, great timing
☐ good pacing & timing
☐ too fast or too slow at times
☐ rhythm felt off

Connection with Students?

- ☐ great connection, used students' names, held group together
- ☐ good connection
- ☐ some students connected, others a little lost
- ☐ felt disconnected

Organization / Planning?

- ☐ teacher available before/after class to chat with students?
- ☐ started/finished on time?
- ☐ was the music appropriate volume and choice?
- ☐ was the mat arrangement / room arrangement appropriate?
- ☐ was the temperature of the room appropriate?

Best thing about the class?

Any areas that felt a little off today?

Other Comments?

CLASS 08 NOTES

Teacher/Studio _____

Class Name: _____   Date of Attendance: _____

Voice Projection:

☐ always clear / easy to hear
☐ mostly clear / easy to hear
☐ some instructions were lost, unclear or confusing
☐ many things were lost (not able to hear)

Physical Assists / Adjustments?

☐ lots of adjustments throughout class
☐ good number of adjustments
☐ some adjustments
☐ lacking adjustments

Energy?

☐ great energy throughout class
☐ good energy
☐ some ups and downs
☐ lacking energy

Rhythm & Pacing?

☐ great pacing, great timing
☐ good pacing & timing
☐ too fast or too slow at times
☐ rhythm felt off

Connection with Students?

- ☐ great connection, used students' names, held group together
- ☐ good connection
- ☐ some students connected, others a little lost
- ☐ felt disconnected

Organization / Planning?

- ☐ teacher available before/after class to chat with students?
- ☐ started/finished on time?
- ☐ was the music appropriate volume and choice?
- ☐ was the mat arrangement / room arrangement appropriate?
- ☐ was the temperature of the room appropriate?

Best thing about the class?

Any areas that felt a little off today?

Other Comments?

CLASS 09 NOTES

Teacher/Studio _____

Class Name: _____ Date of Attendance: _____

Voice Projection:

☐ always clear / easy to hear
☐ mostly clear / easy to hear
☐ some instructions were lost, unclear or confusing
☐ many things were lost (not able to hear)

Physical Assists / Adjustments?

☐ lots of adjustments throughout class
☐ good number of adjustments
☐ some adjustments
☐ lacking adjustments

Energy?

☐ great energy throughout class
☐ good energy
☐ some ups and downs
☐ lacking energy

Rhythm & Pacing?

☐ great pacing, great timing
☐ good pacing & timing
☐ too fast or too slow at times
☐ rhythm felt off

Connection with Students?

- ☐ great connection, used students' names, held group together
- ☐ good connection
- ☐ some students connected, others a little lost
- ☐ felt disconnected

Organization / Planning?

- ☐ teacher available before/after class to chat with students?
- ☐ started/finished on time?
- ☐ was the music appropriate volume and choice?
- ☐ was the mat arrangement / room arrangement appropriate?
- ☐ was the temperature of the room appropriate?

Best thing about the class?

Any areas that felt a little off today?

Other Comments?

CLASS 10 NOTES

Teacher/Studio _____

Class Name: _____ Date of Attendance: _____

Voice Projection:

☐ always clear / easy to hear
☐ mostly clear / easy to hear
☐ some instructions were lost, unclear or confusing
☐ many things were lost (not able to hear)

Physical Assists / Adjustments?

☐ lots of adjustments throughout class
☐ good number of adjustments
☐ some adjustments
☐ lacking adjustments

Energy?

☐ great energy throughout class
☐ good energy
☐ some ups and downs
☐ lacking energy

Rhythm & Pacing?

☐ great pacing, great timing
☐ good pacing & timing
☐ too fast or too slow at times
☐ rhythm felt off

Connection with Students?

- ☐ great connection, used students' names, held group together
- ☐ good connection
- ☐ some students connected, others a little lost
- ☐ felt disconnected

Organization / Planning?

- ☐ teacher available before/after class to chat with students?
- ☐ started/finished on time?
- ☐ was the music appropriate volume and choice?
- ☐ was the mat arrangement / room arrangement appropriate?
- ☐ was the temperature of the room appropriate?

Best thing about the class?

Any areas that felt a little off today?

Other Comments?

CLASS 11 NOTES

Teacher/Studio _____

Class Name: _____ Date of Attendance: _____

Voice Projection:

☐ always clear / easy to hear
☐ mostly clear / easy to hear
☐ some instructions were lost, unclear or confusing
☐ many things were lost (not able to hear)

Physical Assists / Adjustments?

☐ lots of adjustments throughout class
☐ good number of adjustments
☐ some adjustments
☐ lacking adjustments

Energy?

☐ great energy throughout class
☐ good energy
☐ some ups and downs
☐ lacking energy

Rhythm & Pacing?

☐ great pacing, great timing
☐ good pacing & timing
☐ too fast or too slow at times
☐ rhythm felt off

Connection with Students?

- ☐ great connection, used students' names, held group together
- ☐ good connection
- ☐ some students connected, others a little lost
- ☐ felt disconnected

Organization / Planning?

- ☐ teacher available before/after class to chat with students?
- ☐ started/finished on time?
- ☐ was the music appropriate volume and choice?
- ☐ was the mat arrangement / room arrangement appropriate?
- ☐ was the temperature of the room appropriate?

Best thing about the class?

Any areas that felt a little off today?

Other Comments?

CLASS 12 NOTES

Teacher/Studio _____

Class Name: _____ Date of Attendance: _____

Voice Projection:

☐ always clear / easy to hear
☐ mostly clear / easy to hear
☐ some instructions were lost, unclear or confusing
☐ many things were lost (not able to hear)

Physical Assists / Adjustments?

☐ lots of adjustments throughout class
☐ good number of adjustments
☐ some adjustments
☐ lacking adjustments

Energy?

☐ great energy throughout class
☐ good energy
☐ some ups and downs
☐ lacking energy

Rhythm & Pacing?

☐ great pacing, great timing
☐ good pacing & timing
☐ too fast or too slow at times
☐ rhythm felt off

Connection with Students?

- ☐ great connection, used students' names, held group together
- ☐ good connection
- ☐ some students connected, others a little lost
- ☐ felt disconnected

Organization / Planning?

- ☐ teacher available before/after class to chat with students?
- ☐ started/finished on time?
- ☐ was the music appropriate volume and choice?
- ☐ was the mat arrangement / room arrangement appropriate?
- ☐ was the temperature of the room appropriate?

Best thing about the class?

Any areas that felt a little off today?

Other Comments?

CLASS 13 NOTES

Teacher/Studio _____

Class Name: _____ Date of Attendance: _____

Voice Projection:

☐ always clear / easy to hear
☐ mostly clear / easy to hear
☐ some instructions were lost, unclear or confusing
☐ many things were lost (not able to hear)

Physical Assists / Adjustments?

☐ lots of adjustments throughout class
☐ good number of adjustments
☐ some adjustments
☐ lacking adjustments

Energy?

☐ great energy throughout class
☐ good energy
☐ some ups and downs
☐ lacking energy

Rhythm & Pacing?

☐ great pacing, great timing
☐ good pacing & timing
☐ too fast or too slow at times
☐ rhythm felt off

Connection with Students?

- ☐ great connection, used students' names, held group together
- ☐ good connection
- ☐ some students connected, others a little lost
- ☐ felt disconnected

Organization / Planning?

- ☐ teacher available before/after class to chat with students?
- ☐ started/finished on time?
- ☐ was the music appropriate volume and choice?
- ☐ was the mat arrangement / room arrangement appropriate?
- ☐ was the temperature of the room appropriate?

Best thing about the class?

Any areas that felt a little off today?

Other Comments?

CLASS 14 NOTES

Teacher/Studio _____

Class Name: _____ Date of Attendance: _____

Voice Projection:

- ☐ always clear / easy to hear
- ☐ mostly clear / easy to hear
- ☐ some instructions were lost, unclear or confusing
- ☐ many things were lost (not able to hear)

Physical Assists / Adjustments?

- ☐ lots of adjustments throughout class
- ☐ good number of adjustments
- ☐ some adjustments
- ☐ lacking adjustments

Energy?

- ☐ great energy throughout class
- ☐ good energy
- ☐ some ups and downs
- ☐ lacking energy

Rhythm & Pacing?

- ☐ great pacing, great timing
- ☐ good pacing & timing
- ☐ too fast or too slow at times
- ☐ rhythm felt off

Connection with Students?

- ☐ great connection, used students' names, held group together
- ☐ good connection
- ☐ some students connected, others a little lost
- ☐ felt disconnected

Organization / Planning?

- ☐ teacher available before/after class to chat with students?
- ☐ started/finished on time?
- ☐ was the music appropriate volume and choice?
- ☐ was the mat arrangement / room arrangement appropriate?
- ☐ was the temperature of the room appropriate?

Best thing about the class?

Any areas that felt a little off today?

Other Comments?

◤ CLASS 15 NOTES ◥

Teacher/Studio _____

Class Name: _____ Date of Attendance: _____

Voice Projection:

☐ always clear / easy to hear
☐ mostly clear / easy to hear
☐ some instructions were lost, unclear or confusing
☐ many things were lost (not able to hear)

Physical Assists / Adjustments?

☐ lots of adjustments throughout class
☐ good number of adjustments
☐ some adjustments
☐ lacking adjustments

Energy?

☐ great energy throughout class
☐ good energy
☐ some ups and downs
☐ lacking energy

Rhythm & Pacing?

☐ great pacing, great timing
☐ good pacing & timing
☐ too fast or too slow at times
☐ rhythm felt off

Connection with Students?

- ☐ great connection, used students' names, held group together
- ☐ good connection
- ☐ some students connected, others a little lost
- ☐ felt disconnected

Organization / Planning?

- ☐ teacher available before/after class to chat with students?
- ☐ started/finished on time?
- ☐ was the music appropriate volume and choice?
- ☐ was the mat arrangement / room arrangement appropriate?
- ☐ was the temperature of the room appropriate?

Best thing about the class?

Any areas that felt a little off today?

Other Comments?

CLASS 16 NOTES

Teacher/Studio _____

Class Name: _____ Date of Attendance: _____

Voice Projection:

☐ always clear / easy to hear
☐ mostly clear / easy to hear
☐ some instructions were lost, unclear or confusing
☐ many things were lost (not able to hear)

Physical Assists / Adjustments?

☐ lots of adjustments throughout class
☐ good number of adjustments
☐ some adjustments
☐ lacking adjustments

Energy?

☐ great energy throughout class
☐ good energy
☐ some ups and downs
☐ lacking energy

Rhythm & Pacing?

☐ great pacing, great timing
☐ good pacing & timing
☐ too fast or too slow at times
☐ rhythm felt off

Connection with Students?

- ☐ great connection, used students' names, held group together
- ☐ good connection
- ☐ some students connected, others a little lost
- ☐ felt disconnected

Organization / Planning?

- ☐ teacher available before/after class to chat with students?
- ☐ started/finished on time?
- ☐ was the music appropriate volume and choice?
- ☐ was the mat arrangement / room arrangement appropriate?
- ☐ was the temperature of the room appropriate?

Best thing about the class?

Any areas that felt a little off today?

Other Comments?

CLASS 17 NOTES

Teacher/Studio _____

Class Name: _____ Date of Attendance: _____

Voice Projection:

☐ always clear / easy to hear
☐ mostly clear / easy to hear
☐ some instructions were lost, unclear or confusing
☐ many things were lost (not able to hear)

Physical Assists / Adjustments?

☐ lots of adjustments throughout class
☐ good number of adjustments
☐ some adjustments
☐ lacking adjustments

Energy?

☐ great energy throughout class
☐ good energy
☐ some ups and downs
☐ lacking energy

Rhythm & Pacing?

☐ great pacing, great timing
☐ good pacing & timing
☐ too fast or too slow at times
☐ rhythm felt off

Connection with Students?

- ☐ great connection, used students' names, held group together
- ☐ good connection
- ☐ some students connected, others a little lost
- ☐ felt disconnected

Organization / Planning?

- ☐ teacher available before/after class to chat with students?
- ☐ started/finished on time?
- ☐ was the music appropriate volume and choice?
- ☐ was the mat arrangement / room arrangement appropriate?
- ☐ was the temperature of the room appropriate?

Best thing about the class?

Any areas that felt a little off today?

Other Comments?

▶ CLASS 18 NOTES ◀

Teacher/Studio _____

Class Name: _____ Date of Attendance: _____

Voice Projection:

☐ always clear / easy to hear
☐ mostly clear / easy to hear
☐ some instructions were lost, unclear or confusing
☐ many things were lost (not able to hear)

Physical Assists / Adjustments?

☐ lots of adjustments throughout class
☐ good number of adjustments
☐ some adjustments
☐ lacking adjustments

Energy?

☐ great energy throughout class
☐ good energy
☐ some ups and downs
☐ lacking energy

Rhythm & Pacing?

☐ great pacing, great timing
☐ good pacing & timing
☐ too fast or too slow at times
☐ rhythm felt off

Connection with Students?

- ☐ great connection, used students' names, held group together
- ☐ good connection
- ☐ some students connected, others a little lost
- ☐ felt disconnected

Organization / Planning?

- ☐ teacher available before/after class to chat with students?
- ☐ started/finished on time?
- ☐ was the music appropriate volume and choice?
- ☐ was the mat arrangement / room arrangement appropriate?
- ☐ was the temperature of the room appropriate?

Best thing about the class?

Any areas that felt a little off today?

Other Comments?

CLASS 19 NOTES

Teacher/Studio _____

Class Name: _____ Date of Attendance: _____

Voice Projection:

☐ always clear / easy to hear
☐ mostly clear / easy to hear
☐ some instructions were lost, unclear or confusing
☐ many things were lost (not able to hear)

Physical Assists / Adjustments?

☐ lots of adjustments throughout class
☐ good number of adjustments
☐ some adjustments
☐ lacking adjustments

Energy?

☐ great energy throughout class
☐ good energy
☐ some ups and downs
☐ lacking energy

Rhythm & Pacing?

☐ great pacing, great timing
☐ good pacing & timing
☐ too fast or too slow at times
☐ rhythm felt off

Connection with Students?

- ☐ great connection, used students' names, held group together
- ☐ good connection
- ☐ some students connected, others a little lost
- ☐ felt disconnected

Organization / Planning?

- ☐ teacher available before/after class to chat with students?
- ☐ started/finished on time?
- ☐ was the music appropriate volume and choice?
- ☐ was the mat arrangement / room arrangement appropriate?
- ☐ was the temperature of the room appropriate?

Best thing about the class?

Any areas that felt a little off today?

Other Comments?

CLASS 20 NOTES

Teacher/Studio _____

Class Name: _____ Date of Attendance: _____

Voice Projection:

☐ always clear / easy to hear
☐ mostly clear / easy to hear
☐ some instructions were lost, unclear or confusing
☐ many things were lost (not able to hear)

Physical Assists / Adjustments?

☐ lots of adjustments throughout class
☐ good number of adjustments
☐ some adjustments
☐ lacking adjustments

Energy?

☐ great energy throughout class
☐ good energy
☐ some ups and downs
☐ lacking energy

Rhythm & Pacing?

☐ great pacing, great timing
☐ good pacing & timing
☐ too fast or too slow at times
☐ rhythm felt off

Connection with Students?

- ☐ great connection, used students' names, held group together
- ☐ good connection
- ☐ some students connected, others a little lost
- ☐ felt disconnected

Organization / Planning?

- ☐ teacher available before/after class to chat with students?
- ☐ started/finished on time?
- ☐ was the music appropriate volume and choice?
- ☐ was the mat arrangement / room arrangement appropriate?
- ☐ was the temperature of the room appropriate?

Best thing about the class?

Any areas that felt a little off today?

Other Comments?

CLASS 21 NOTES

Teacher/Studio _____

Class Name: _____ Date of Attendance: _____

Voice Projection:

☐ always clear / easy to hear
☐ mostly clear / easy to hear
☐ some instructions were lost, unclear or confusing
☐ many things were lost (not able to hear)

Physical Assists / Adjustments?

☐ lots of adjustments throughout class
☐ good number of adjustments
☐ some adjustments
☐ lacking adjustments

Energy?

☐ great energy throughout class
☐ good energy
☐ some ups and downs
☐ lacking energy

Rhythm & Pacing?

☐ great pacing, great timing
☐ good pacing & timing
☐ too fast or too slow at times
☐ rhythm felt off

Connection with Students?

- ☐ great connection, used students' names, held group together
- ☐ good connection
- ☐ some students connected, others a little lost
- ☐ felt disconnected

Organization / Planning?

- ☐ teacher available before/after class to chat with students?
- ☐ started/finished on time?
- ☐ was the music appropriate volume and choice?
- ☐ was the mat arrangement / room arrangement appropriate?
- ☐ was the temperature of the room appropriate?

Best thing about the class?

Any areas that felt a little off today?

Other Comments?

CLASS 22 NOTES

Teacher/Studio _____

Class Name: _____ Date of Attendance: _____

Voice Projection:

☐ always clear / easy to hear
☐ mostly clear / easy to hear
☐ some instructions were lost, unclear or confusing
☐ many things were lost (not able to hear)

Physical Assists / Adjustments?

☐ lots of adjustments throughout class
☐ good number of adjustments
☐ some adjustments
☐ lacking adjustments

Energy?

☐ great energy throughout class
☐ good energy
☐ some ups and downs
☐ lacking energy

Rhythm & Pacing?

☐ great pacing, great timing
☐ good pacing & timing
☐ too fast or too slow at times
☐ rhythm felt off

Connection with Students?

- ☐ great connection, used students' names, held group together
- ☐ good connection
- ☐ some students connected, others a little lost
- ☐ felt disconnected

Organization / Planning?

- ☐ teacher available before/after class to chat with students?
- ☐ started/finished on time?
- ☐ was the music appropriate volume and choice?
- ☐ was the mat arrangement / room arrangement appropriate?
- ☐ was the temperature of the room appropriate?

Best thing about the class?

Any areas that felt a little off today?

Other Comments?

CLASS 23 NOTES

Teacher/Studio _____

Class Name: _____   Date of Attendance: _____

Voice Projection:

☐ always clear / easy to hear
☐ mostly clear / easy to hear
☐ some instructions were lost, unclear or confusing
☐ many things were lost (not able to hear)

Physical Assists / Adjustments?

☐ lots of adjustments throughout class
☐ good number of adjustments
☐ some adjustments
☐ lacking adjustments

Energy?

☐ great energy throughout class
☐ good energy
☐ some ups and downs
☐ lacking energy

Rhythm & Pacing?

☐ great pacing, great timing
☐ good pacing & timing
☐ too fast or too slow at times
☐ rhythm felt off

Connection with Students?

- ☐ great connection, used students' names, held group together
- ☐ good connection
- ☐ some students connected, others a little lost
- ☐ felt disconnected

Organization / Planning?

- ☐ teacher available before/after class to chat with students?
- ☐ started/finished on time?
- ☐ was the music appropriate volume and choice?
- ☐ was the mat arrangement / room arrangement appropriate?
- ☐ was the temperature of the room appropriate?

Best thing about the class?

Any areas that felt a little off today?

Other Comments?

CLASS 24 NOTES

Teacher/Studio _____

Class Name: _____ Date of Attendance: _____

Voice Projection:

☐ always clear / easy to hear
☐ mostly clear / easy to hear
☐ some instructions were lost, unclear or confusing
☐ many things were lost (not able to hear)

Physical Assists / Adjustments?

☐ lots of adjustments throughout class
☐ good number of adjustments
☐ some adjustments
☐ lacking adjustments

Energy?

☐ great energy throughout class
☐ good energy
☐ some ups and downs
☐ lacking energy

Rhythm & Pacing?

☐ great pacing, great timing
☐ good pacing & timing
☐ too fast or too slow at times
☐ rhythm felt off

Connection with Students?

- ☐ great connection, used students' names, held group together
- ☐ good connection
- ☐ some students connected, others a little lost
- ☐ felt disconnected

Organization / Planning?

- ☐ teacher available before/after class to chat with students?
- ☐ started/finished on time?
- ☐ was the music appropriate volume and choice?
- ☐ was the mat arrangement / room arrangement appropriate?
- ☐ was the temperature of the room appropriate?

Best thing about the class?

Any areas that felt a little off today?

Other Comments?

CLASS 25 NOTES

Teacher/Studio _____

Class Name: _____ Date of Attendance: _____

Voice Projection:

☐ always clear / easy to hear
☐ mostly clear / easy to hear
☐ some instructions were lost, unclear or confusing
☐ many things were lost (not able to hear)

Physical Assists / Adjustments?

☐ lots of adjustments throughout class
☐ good number of adjustments
☐ some adjustments
☐ lacking adjustments

Energy?

☐ great energy throughout class
☐ good energy
☐ some ups and downs
☐ lacking energy

Rhythm & Pacing?

☐ great pacing, great timing
☐ good pacing & timing
☐ too fast or too slow at times
☐ rhythm felt off

Connection with Students?

- ☐ great connection, used students' names, held group together
- ☐ good connection
- ☐ some students connected, others a little lost
- ☐ felt disconnected

Organization / Planning?

- ☐ teacher available before/after class to chat with students?
- ☐ started/finished on time?
- ☐ was the music appropriate volume and choice?
- ☐ was the mat arrangement / room arrangement appropriate?
- ☐ was the temperature of the room appropriate?

Best thing about the class?

Any areas that felt a little off today?

Other Comments?

If you want to test your memory, try to recall what you were worrying about one year ago today.

— E. Joseph Cossman

PRACTICE TEACHING & STUDENT REVIEWS

Practice teaching with friends, family and volunteers is a crucial part of your learning experience. At YOGABODY, we're here to train industry leaders, and leaders welcome feedback to learn and grow as professionals.

Here's How this Process Works:

Step 1. Teach a practice class with friends, family or volunteers.

Step 2. Have at least 1 student review your class using this form.

Step 3. Share this feedback with your teaching mentor.

STUDENT REVIEWS — 1 OF 5

Thanks for taking the time to share your feedback on my class today. Quite simply, I'd love to know how you think it went?

1. How was my voice projection?

2. How were my adjustments and assists?

3. Did you think my energy level was appropriate?

4. What did you think of my rhythm & pacing?

5. Would you take this class again?

6. Any suggestions based on your experience?

7. Other Comments?

STUDENT REVIEWS — 2 OF 5

Thanks for taking the time to share your feedback on my class today. Quite simply, I'd love to know how you think it went?

1. How was my voice projection?

2. How were my adjustments and assists?

3. Did you think my energy level was appropriate?

4. What did you think of my rhythm & pacing?

5. Would you take this class again?

6. Any suggestions based on your experience?

7. Other Comments?

STUDENT REVIEWS — 3 OF 5

Thanks for taking the time to share your feedback on my class today. Quite simply, I'd love to know how you think it went?

1. How was my voice projection?

2. How were my adjustments and assists?

3. Did you think my energy level was appropriate?

4. What did you think of my rhythm & pacing?

5. Would you take this class again?

6. Any suggestions based on your experience?

7. Other Comments?

STUDENT REVIEWS — 4 OF 5

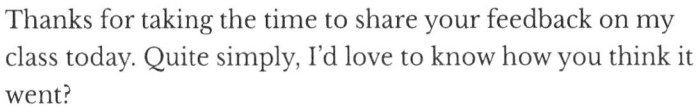

Thanks for taking the time to share your feedback on my class today. Quite simply, I'd love to know how you think it went?

1. How was my voice projection?

2. How were my adjustments and assists?

3. Did you think my energy level was appropriate?

4. What did you think of my rhythm & pacing?

5. Would you take this class again?

6. Any suggestions based on your experience?

7. Other Comments?

STUDENT REVIEWS — 5 OF 5

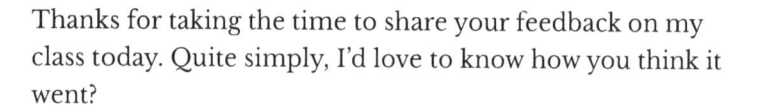

Thanks for taking the time to share your feedback on my class today. Quite simply, I'd love to know how you think it went?

1. How was my voice projection?

2. How were my adjustments and assists?

3. Did you think my energy level was appropriate?

4. What did you think of my rhythm & pacing?

5. Would you take this class again?

6. Any suggestions based on your experience?

7. Other Comments?

YOGABODY STYLE ORIGINS

In the yoga community, there is disagreement about when yoga as we know it today first began. Some say thousands of years ago, some say around one hundred years ago. Most of this confusion occurs when people mix up the philosophical tradition of yoga with the modern practice of Hatha Yoga, the physical practices of posture and breath work.

Yoga is one of the 6 systems of Indian philosophy, but the yoga philosophical tradition and the physical yoga we practice at YOGABODY have almost nothing in common except the name, yoga.

At YOGABODY, we seek to democratize yoga and we teach these mind-body practices free of any fixed philosophical or religious context. We respect and accept all philosophical, spiritual, and religions of the world, but we do not teach or associate with one as a group; instead, our YOGABODY students include everyone from spiritual philosophers to atheists, Jews, Christians, and Muslims.

All beliefs, all backgrounds, and all positive people are welcome at YOGABODY. We're here to support you with your health, not to tell you how or what to believe. With that in mind, the yoga we practice can be clearly traced back to the 1930's in Mysore, India to a teacher named, Krishnamacharya.

Arguably the most influential yoga teacher to ever live, Krishnamacharya was commissioned by the king of Mysore to teach yoga locally, mostly to young boys. From the few photos and accounts available from that time, it's very clear that this yoga program was very much focused on posture and breath—not religion or philosophy.

While people have certainly done some form of yoga postures forever, the idea of a sequenced, athletic series of poses linked together with breath seems to have been pioneered by Krishnamacharya and planted the seed for the modern yoga revolution.

Whatever the mind of man can conceive and believe, it can achieve.

– Napoleon Hill

MISC. NOTES

~~The End~~
The Beginning

YOGABODY Naturals LLC
302 Washington St #150-6920
San Diego, CA 92103
www.YogaBody.com
help@yogabody.com | (310) 294-3550

CPSIA information can be obtained
at www.ICGtesting.com
Printed in the USA
FSHW020104120520
69895FS